NATURAL REMEDY FOR JOINT PAIN

Home Remedies for Joint Pain Relief

CHRIS WILLIAM

copyright

Table of content

INTRODUCTION

Joint pain is a frustrating and often debilitating condition that can affect anyone at any age. For me, it started when I was in my mid-thirties. I was an avid runner and enjoyed playing tennis and walking my dogs in the park. I was fit and healthy, but one day, out of nowhere, I started experiencing severe pain in my hips and knees.

At first, I thought it was just a normal ache or soreness that would go away on its own. However, the pain persisted and I started to worry. I tried over-the-counter pain medications, but they didn't do much to relieve the discomfort. I considered going to my doctor, but I was worried that they might think I was exaggerating and prescribe me a heavy-duty medication that I didn't need.

I decided to take matters into my own hands and started researching natural remedies for joint pain. I soon discovered that there were many natural remedies out there that could help me manage my pain and potentially even get rid of it altogether. I started taking daily supplements of fish oil, glucosamine, and chondroitin. I also started doing gentle exercises and stretches to help strengthen my muscles and joints.

At first, I didn't notice much of a difference, but I kept at it. Over time, I started to see a gradual improvement. The pain slowly began to fade away and I was able to get back to my regular activities without any discomfort. I was so relieved and thankful that I had found a way to overcome joint pain without the need for heavy-duty medications.

The joint pain had taken a toll on my life in more ways than one. It had been a constant reminder of my own mortality and fragility. It had also taken away some of my joy and motivation to do the things I loved. Now, with the help of natural remedies, I was able to reclaim my life and find joy again.

My experience with joint pain has taught me a lot of valuable lessons. It has made me realize that it is possible to manage and overcome chronic pain without relying too heavily on medication. It has also made me appreciate the importance of taking care of my body and mind.

This is just the beginning of my journey. In the next chapter of my story, I'll discuss how I've been able to maintain my health and keep my joint pain under control. I'll share my experiences

with natural treatments and how they've helped me stay healthy and active. I'll also discuss some tips for those who may be considering natural remedies for joint pain. Join me on my journey to discover how natural remedies can help you overcome joint pain.

CHAPTER ONE

WHAT IS JOINT PAIN?

Joint pain (also referred to as arthralgia) is a very common symptom that affects millions of people worldwide. It can be caused by a variety of conditions, including arthritis, bursitis, tendinitis, muscle strain, gout, and other injuries. Joint pain is typically characterized by aching,

stiffness, and/or soreness in the affected joint or joints. It can range from mild discomfort to severe and debilitating pain. Other symptoms may include swelling, redness, or warmth in the joint area, as well as decreased range of motion. Treatment for joint pain depends on the underlying cause but may include pain medications, lifestyle modifications, physical therapy, and injections.

Joint pain is caused by a variety of conditions and can affect any joint in the body. Common causes include:

1. Arthritis

Arthritis is a condition that affects the joints, causing pain and inflammation. It can be caused by a variety of factors, including age, genetic factors, and lifestyle. Depending on the specific type of arthritis, the symptoms can range from mild to severe. Joint pain, stiffness, swelling, and decreased range of motion are all common symptoms associated with arthritis.

Joint pain is the most common symptom associated with arthritis. This pain is caused by inflammation, which is the body's natural response to injury or irritation. When the joints are inflamed, the tissues that make up the joint can become damaged, resulting in pain. Additionally, the inflamed tissues may accumulate fluid, causing swelling and further inflammation.

The inflammation that occurs in the joints can also lead to stiffness, as the tissues become less flexible. This can make it difficult to move the joint, leading to decreased range of motion. As arthritis progresses, the joint can become increasingly stiff and painful, making it difficult to perform normal activities.

In addition to inflammation, arthritis can also lead to the formation of bone spurs. These bony growths can develop on the edges of the joints, leading to further pain and stiffness. As the condition progresses, these bone spurs can make it difficult to move the joint, leading to even more pain and decreased range of motion.

Finally, arthritis can also lead to the breakdown of cartilage. Cartilage is a substance that helps to cushion the joint and allows for smooth movement. When the cartilage is broken down, the joint can become prone to pain and stiffness.

Overall, arthritis can cause a variety of symptoms, including joint pain, stiffness, swelling, decreased range of motion, and the formation of bone spurs. The severity of the symptoms can vary depending on the type of arthritis and the stage of the condition. Treatment for arthritis can involve lifestyle changes, medications, and physical therapy, and can help reduce pain and improve mobility.

2. Bursitis

Bursitis is an inflammatory condition of the bursa, a fluid-filled sac located near joints in the body. It is a common cause of joint pain and can affect a variety of different parts of the body, including the shoulders, elbows, hips, knees, and heels. Bursitis is often caused by overuse, trauma, or infection.

When bursitis occurs, the bursa becomes inflamed, leading to swelling and pain at the joint. In some cases, there may also be redness, warmth, and tenderness to the touch. The pain can range from mild to severe and is usually worse when the affected joint is used. It may also be accompanied by a feeling of stiffness, making it difficult to move the joint.

The main cause of bursitis is overuse of the joint. This can cause the bursa to become irritated and inflamed, leading to pain and swelling. Overuse can be due to repetitive motions, such as those involved in certain sports, or from holding a joint in a certain position for too long. In addition, direct trauma to the joint, such as a fall or blow, can also cause bursitis.

Infection can also be a cause of bursitis. Bacteria, fungi, and viruses can all cause inflammation of the bursa, leading to pain and swelling. Bacterial infections are the most common cause of bursitis and can be spread through skin-to-skin contact or contact with contaminated surfaces.

Bursitis can be treated with rest, ice, compression, and elevation (RICE). This can help reduce swelling and pain and allow the bursa to heal. Non-steroidal anti-inflammatory drugs (NSAIDs) such as ibuprofen or naproxen may also be used to reduce pain and swelling. In some cases, a corticosteroid injection may be used to reduce inflammation.

In more severe cases of bursitis, surgery may be necessary to remove the inflamed bursa. This can alleviate pain and allow the joint to return to full function. Physical therapy may also be recommended to improve flexibility and strength in the joint.

Bursitis can cause joint pain that can range from mild to severe. It is usually caused by overuse or trauma to the joint, but can also be caused by infection.

3. Tendinitis

Tendinitis is an inflammation of a tendon, the tough fibrous cords that attach muscle to bone. It is an overuse injury that occurs when the tendon is overworked, strained, or injured. Tendinitis can cause joint pain, weakness, and swelling around the affected joint.

The most common causes of tendinitis are repetitive movements, such as those that occur during sports or jobs that require repetitive motions. For example, running, jumping, and lifting can put excess strain on the tendons that attach to the knee, hips, elbows, and shoulders. Overuse of these tendons can lead to inflammation and irritation, resulting in joint pain.

Tendinitis can also be caused by direct trauma to the joint or tendon, such as a fall or a blow to the area. This can cause inflammation and irritation of the tendon, leading to joint pain and stiffness.

When tendinitis is the cause of joint pain, the pain is usually felt near the affected joint. This is because the tendon is inflamed and irritated, leading to pain that can range from mild to severe. Pain can become worse with movement, such as bending or extending the affected joint. The affected joint may also be tender to the touch, and there may be swelling in the area.

Treatment of tendinitis includes rest, ice, compression, and elevation of the affected joint. Anti-inflammatory medications can also be used to reduce inflammation and pain. In severe cases, surgery may be necessary to repair the tendon.

Physical therapy can also be beneficial in the treatment of tendinitis. A physical therapist can help strengthen the affected area and improve the range of motion. Exercises to stretch and strengthen the affected joint can help reduce pain and improve the range of motion.

Although tendinitis may cause joint pain, it is important to get an accurate diagnosis from a doctor or physical therapist. This will help ensure that the correct treatment plan is used to reduce joint pain and improve the range of motion.

4. Muscle strain

Muscle strain, also known as a pulled muscle, occurs when the fibers in a muscle are stretched or torn. This can happen as a result of overuse, improper form during physical activity, or a sudden injury. When a muscle strain occurs, it can cause pain, weakness, and difficulty moving the affected muscle. If the muscle strain is severe, it can also lead to joint pain.

Joint pain is a common symptom of muscle strain because the muscles and tendons that surround a joint play a crucial role in supporting and stabilizing the joint. When a muscle is strained, it can become inflamed and swollen, which can put pressure on the tendons and ligaments that connect the muscle to the bone. This pressure can cause pain and inflammation in the joint, making it difficult to move.

Another way that muscle strain can cause joint pain is through muscle imbalances. When a muscle is strained, it can become weaker and less flexible, which can lead to an imbalance in the muscles around the joint. This can cause the other muscles to work harder to compensate, which can lead to overuse and pain in the joint.

Muscle strain can also cause joint pain by affecting the alignment of the joint. When a muscle is strained, it can pull on the bone it is attached to, which can cause the joint to become misaligned. This can lead to pain and discomfort as the joint is forced to move in an unnatural position.

In addition to causing joint pain, muscle strain can also lead to other problems such as stiffness, muscle spasms, and muscle weakness. The severity of muscle strain can vary, and treatment will depend on the extent of the injury. Rest and physical therapy are often recommended to help the muscle heal and regain strength and flexibility. In severe cases, surgery may be necessary to repair the damaged muscle.

In summary, muscle strain can cause joint pain through several mechanisms: putting pressure on tendons and ligaments that connect muscle to bone, muscle imbalances, and affecting the alignment of the joint. It is important to take steps to prevent muscle strain, such as warming up properly before physical activity and using proper form during exercise. If you do experience a muscle strain, it is important to rest and seek treatment to help the muscle heal and prevent further injury.

Gout:

A gout is a form of arthritis caused by the buildup of uric acid crystals in the joints. These crystals can cause inflammation, pain, and stiffness in the affected joints. The most common joint affected by gout is the big toe, but it can also affect the ankles, knees, elbows, wrists, and fingers.

Uric acid is a waste product that is created when the body breaks down purines, which are found in many foods, including red meat, organ meats, and seafood. In some people, the body produces too much uric acid or is not able to effectively remove it through the kidneys. This can cause the uric acid to crystallize and deposit in the joints and surrounding tissue.

The symptoms of gout typically appear suddenly and can include severe pain, redness, and swelling in the affected joint. The joint may also feel warm to the touch and be stiff and difficult to move. The pain can be so severe that it makes it difficult to walk or even sleep. These symptoms usually last for a few days to a week but can recur if the underlying cause of the gout is not treated.

The diagnosis of gout is typically made based on the symptoms and a physical examination. A blood test can also be done to measure the level of uric acid in the blood. If gout is suspected, a sample of fluid from the affected joint may also be taken to be examined for uric acid crystals.

Treatment for gout typically involves medication to reduce pain and inflammation, as well as to lower the level of uric acid in the blood. Non-steroidal anti-inflammatory drugs (NSAIDs) such as ibuprofen and naproxen are commonly used to relieve pain and inflammation. Colchicine, a medication specifically designed to treat gout, may also be prescribed.

Other medications, such as allopurinol, febuxostat, or probenecid, can help to lower the level of uric acid in the blood and reduce the risk of future gout attacks. These medications can take several weeks to take effect, and are usualprescribed for long-term use.

In addition to medication, lifestyle changes can also help to manage gout. Avoiding foods that are high in purines, such as red meat, organ meats, and seafood, can help to lower the risk of gout attacks. Drinking plenty of water and staying hydrated can also help to flush excess uric acid out of the body.

Gout can be a debilitating and painful condition, but it is treatable with the right combination of medication, lifestyle changes, and ongoing management. With the right treatment, people with gout can reduce their risk of future attacks and improve their overall quality of life.

Injuries:

Joint pain is a common symptom of injury, which can occur in any joint in the body but is most commonly felt in the knees, hips, shoulders, and wrists. Joints are the points where two or more bones come together, and they are held together by strong connective tissue called ligaments. Joints also have a cushioning layer called cartilage, which helps to absorb shock and reduce friction between bones.

Injuries to joints can occur in several ways. The most common cause of joint pain is a sprain, which occurs when a ligament is stretched or torn. This can happen from a sudden impact, such as a fall or a blow to the joint, or from overuse, such as repetitive motions in sports or work. Sprains can cause pain, swelling, and stiffness in the joint, and in severe cases, they can also cause a loss of range of

motion.

CHAPTER TWO

NATURAL REMEDIES FOR JOINT PAIN

Joint pain is a common and uncomfortable experience for many people. It can range from a dull ache to a sharp, burning sensation and can be caused by a variety of issues from age-related degeneration to inflammation. Fortunately, there are many natural remedies that can help

reduce joint pain and improve overall joint health. These natural remedies can include lifestyle changes such as changing diet, exercising regularly, and reducing stress levels as well as supplements, herbs, and essential oils that can help reduce inflammation and ease the pain. This article will provide an overview of some of the most effective natural remedies for joint pain, including how they work and how to use them safely and effectively. Additionally, the safety of using natural remedies for joint pain will be discussed, as well as other potential treatments.

By the end of this chapter, you will have a better understanding of how to safely and effectively use natural remedies for joint pain.

DIET AND NUTRITION

Diet and nutrition can play an important role in managing joint pain. Some of the nutrients that can be beneficial for joint health include omega-3 fatty acids, vitamin C, vitamin D, and glucosamine. In addition to consuming foods that are rich in these nutrients, avoiding certain foods can also help to manage joint pain. For example, avoiding processed and fried foods, as well as foods with added sugar, can help reduce inflammation and provide relief from joint pain.

FOODS TO INCLUDE

1. Omega-3 Fatty Acids

Omega-3 fatty acids are essential fatty acids that are important for overall health. They are known to be beneficial for joint pain, as they are anti-inflammatory and can help reduce inflammation and swelling in the joints. Omega-3 fatty acids also help to lubricate the joints

and improve joint flexibility, which can reduce pain and stiffness associated with osteoarthritis. Studies have also shown that omega-3 fatty acids are effective at reducing morning stiffness and pain in those with rheumatoid arthritis. Additionally, omega-3 fatty acids can help reduce inflammation and pain associated with other types of joint pain, such as bursitis and tendinitis. The best sources of omega-3 fatty acids are fatty fish, such as salmon, mackerel, and sardines, as well as walnuts, chia seeds, and flaxseeds.

Incorporating omega-3 fatty acids into your diet is an effective way to reduce joint pain and improve overall joint health. Eating a diet rich in omega-3 fatty acids can help reduce inflammation, improve joint flexibility, and reduce pain. Additionally, research has shown that taking omega-3 supplements may also be effective in reducing joint pain and inflammation. If you are considering taking omega-3 supplements, it is important to consult with your healthcare provider to ensure that the supplement is right for you.

Overall, omega-3 fatty acids are beneficial for reducing joint pain and inflammation. Eating a diet rich in omega-3 fatty acids and considering taking a supplement can help reduce joint pain and improve overall joint health.

2. Vitamin C

Vitamin C is an essential vitamin that plays an important role in protecting the body from damage caused by free radicals. It is also an important factor in the production of collagen, which is necessary for the formation of healthy bones, cartilage, and connective tissues. Vitamin C can help to reduce joint pain and stiffness by improving the structure of collagen and promoting the repair of damaged cartilage. Vitamin C can also help to reduce inflammation, which is often the cause of joint pain. Additionally, Vitamin C helps to improve the absorption of iron, which is necessary for the production of healthy joint tissues. Lastly, Vitamin C helps to boost the immune system, which can help to reduce inflammation and reduce the severity of joint pain.

Overall, Vitamin C plays an important role in reducing joint pain and stiffness. It helps to improve the structure of collagen, reduce inflammation, and promote the absorption of iron and immune system strength. For these reasons, it is important to include Vitamin C in your diet if you are experiencing joint pain.

Foods rich in Vitamin C include citrus fruits, peppers, dark leafy greens, and cruciferous vegetables. Supplementation is also an option for those who are unable to get enough Vitamin C from their diet. By consuming Vitamin C regularly, you can help to reduce joint pain and improve the overall health of your joints.

Vitamin C is a powerful tool in the fight against joint pain. It helps to reduce inflammation and promote the production of collagen, which is necessary for healthy bones, cartilage, and connective tissues. Vitamin C can also improve the absorption of iron, which is important for joint health. Additionally, Vitamin C can help to boost the immune system, which can help to reduce inflammation and reduce the severity of joint pain. It is important to include Vitamin C in your diet, either through dietary sources or through supplementation, to help reduce joint pain and improve joint health.

3. Vitamin D

Vitamin D is an essential vitamin that helps regulate calcium absorption, which is necessary for healthy bones and teeth. It is also essential for optimal immune system function, and it may help reduce the risk of some chronic diseases such as cancer and heart disease. Vitamin D is also known to help reduce joint pain, especially for those suffering from arthritis. It helps to reduce inflammation, which can be a major contributing factor to joint pain. Vitamin D helps to strengthen the bones and improve their flexibility, which can help to reduce the discomfort in the joints caused by arthritis. Additionally, Vitamin D helps to regulate hormones and

neurotransmitters, which can help to reduce pain and improve mood. For individuals living with chronic joint pain, increasing their Vitamin D intake can be an effective way to reduce their pain and improve their overall quality of life.

Getting enough Vitamin D can be difficult, as it is not naturally produced in the body and must be obtained through dietary sources or supplements. Foods like dairy, eggs, fish, and mushrooms are all good sources of Vitamin D, and many foods are also fortified with it.

Additionally, spending time in the sun is a great way to get Vitamin D, as the body produces it in response to UV light exposure. For those who are unable to get enough Vitamin D through their diet or sunlight, taking a supplement is a great option. However, it is important to ensure that you are not taking too much, as excessive levels of Vitamin D can be toxic.

In conclusion, Vitamin D is an essential vitamin that helps to reduce joint pain associated with arthritis. It helps to reduce inflammation, strengthen the bones, and regulate hormones and neurotransmitters, all of which can help to reduce pain and improve quality of life. Getting

enough Vitamin D can be difficult, so it is important to ensure that you are getting enough through your diet or supplements.

4. Glucosamine

Glucosamine is a naturally occurring substance found in the body that helps to maintain healthy cartilage, the tissue that cushions the joints. It is often taken as a supplement to help relieve joint pain and stiffness associated with arthritis. Studies have found that glucosamine may help

reduce joint pain and improve joint function in people with mild to moderate osteoarthritis. It is thought to work by helping to maintain the structure and integrity of cartilage, which may reduce inflammation and pain associated with arthritis. Additionally, some studies have

suggested that glucosamine may help reduce the progression of osteoarthritis, although more research is needed to confirm these findings. In general, most people tolerate glucosamine well, although some may experience mild side effects such as nausea, headaches, and heartburn. It is important to speak with a doctor before taking glucosamine, as it may interact with certain medications.

Glucosamine is an important supplement for those who suffer from joint pain and stiffness due to arthritis. However, it is important to note that it is not a cure for arthritis and that pain relief will likely be gradual. Additionally, it is important to combine glucosamine with other treatments such as physical therapy and diet modifications to optimize results.

Overall, glucosamine is a safe, natural supplement that may help reduce joint pain and stiffness associated with osteoarthritis. While more research is needed to fully understand its potential benefits, it may be worth a try for those who suffer from joint pain and stiffness due to arthritis.

FOODS TO AVOID

1. Processed and Fried Foods

Processed and fried foods should be avoided for joint pain, as they can cause inflammation. These foods are high in unhealthy fats that can cause inflammation in the body, which can lead to joint pain. In addition, fried and processed foods often contain chemical additives and preservatives that can also increase inflammation. Eating these foods can also lead to weight gain, which can put extra strain and stress on the joints, resulting in even more pain. Instead, it is better to focus on eating a healthy, balanced diet that is rich in fresh fruits and vegetables, lean proteins, and whole grains. These foods are anti-inflammatory and provide the body with essential nutrients that can help reduce joint pain.

In addition to avoiding processed and fried foods, it is important to stay active and get regular physical activity. Exercise can help keep joints flexible and strong, and can help reduce joint pain. Stretching and low-impact activities, such as walking, swimming, or yoga, are especially beneficial for joint pain. It is important to talk to a doctor before beginning any kind of exercise program.

Overall, avoiding processed and fried foods is one of the best ways to help reduce joint pain. These foods can cause inflammation and can add extra strain to the joints. It is better to focus on eating a healthy, balanced diet and getting regular physical activity to help reduce joint pain.

2. Foods with Added Sugar

Consuming foods with added sugar can have a negative impact on our joints, leading to pain and inflammation. Added sugar, also known as free sugar, is the sugar that is added to food during processing and preparation, as opposed to the natural sugar found in fruits and vegetables.

One of the main ways that added sugar can contribute to joint pain is through its inflammatory properties. When we consume sugar, our body releases a hormone called insulin, which helps to regulate blood sugar levels. However, when we consume too much sugar, our body's insulin response can become overactive, leading to chronic inflammation. This inflammation can cause damage to the joints, leading to conditions such as osteoarthritis.

In addition to inflammation, consuming too much-added sugar can also lead to weight gain. Being overweight or obese puts extra stress on the joints, especially in the hips, knees, and ankles. This extra stress can lead to pain and inflammation in these joints, as well as an increased risk of developing osteoarthritis.

Furthermore, high sugar intake has been linked to the development of type 2 diabetes, which can also contribute to joint pain. Diabetes is a metabolic disorder that affects the way our body uses sugar, and when it is not managed properly, it can cause damage to the nerves and blood vessels, leading to pain and numbness in the feet and legs. In some cases, this pain can also affect the hips, knees, and hands.

Another way that added sugar can contribute to joint pain is by disrupting the balance of certain nutrients in our bodies. When we consume too much sugar, it can displace other important nutrients that our joints need to stay healthy, such as calcium and vitamin D. Calcium is essential for maintaining strong bones and joints, and vitamin D helps our body to absorb calcium. When we consume too much sugar, it can displace these important nutrients, leading to weaker bones and joints, which can contribute to pain and inflammation.

It is important to note that added sugar can be found in many types of food and drinks, not just desserts. Many processed foods, such as bread, cereal, and pasta sauce, contain added sugar. Even some foods that are marketed as "healthy" or "low-fat" can contain added sugar. Therefore, it's crucial to be aware of the added sugar content in the foods we consume and to read the labels carefully.

To avoid the negative impact of added sugar on our joints, it's recommended to limit or avoid foods with added sugar. Instead, we should focus on consuming a diet rich in whole foods.

3. Alcohol

Alcohol consumption can have a negative impact on joint health and can exacerbate symptoms of joint pain.

One of the primary ways that alcohol can affect joint pain is through its impact on inflammation. When consumed in large quantities, alcohol can increase inflammation throughout the body. This can lead to increased pain and stiffness in the joints, making it more difficult to move and perform daily activities. Additionally, alcohol can also inhibit the body's ability to repair damaged tissue, which can prolong the healing time for injuries or conditions that affect the joints.

Another way that alcohol can affect joint health is through its impact on bone density. Regular alcohol consumption can lead to decreased bone density, which can increase the risk of bone fractures and other injuries. This is particularly concerning for individuals who are already at risk for osteoporosis or other conditions that affect bone health.

Alcohol can also have an impact on weight, and excessive weight can put additional stress on the joints. This can lead to increased pain and inflammation, and can also make it more difficult to maintain mobility and independence.

Furthermore, excessive alcohol consumption can lead to liver damage and other health problems, which can have a negative impact on overall well-being. This can make it more difficult for individuals to manage their joint pain and other symptoms, and can also make it harder for them to engage in physical activity and other treatments that can help to alleviate joint pain.

In conclusion, alcohol consumption can have a negative impact on joint health and can exacerbate symptoms of joint pain. It's important for individuals who experience joint pain to be mindful of their alcohol consumption and to speak with their healthcare provider about any concerns they may have. Additionally, it's also important to maintain a healthy weight, exercise regularly, and follow a well-balanced diet in order to keep the joints healthy.

4. Dairy Products

Dairy products are a common dietary staple, but those experiencing joint pain may want to consider limiting their consumption. There are a few reasons why avoiding or limiting dairy products may be beneficial for joint health.

One reason is that dairy products contain a protein called casein, which has been shown to promote inflammation in the body. Inflammation is a key contributor to joint pain and stiffness, and consuming dairy products can exacerbate these symptoms. Additionally, many individuals may be lactose intolerant, which means they have difficulty digesting the sugar found in milk and dairy products. This can lead to bloating, gas, and abdominal pain, which can also contribute to joint pain.

Another reason to avoid dairy products for joint pain is that they are high in saturated fat. Consuming too much-saturated fat can lead to weight gain, which can put additional stress on the joints and make the pain worse. Additionally, research suggests that a diet high in saturated fat may increase the risk of developing osteoarthritis, a condition that affects the joints and causes pain and stiffness.

Dairy products are also known to be one of the most common food allergens, and an allergic reaction can cause inflammation in the body. Allergic reactions can manifest in various ways, including joint pain and stiffness.

Moreover, some studies have found that consuming dairy products may increase the risk of developing gout, a type of arthritis that causes severe pain and inflammation in the joints. This is because dairy products are high in purines, which can increase the levels of uric acid in the blood, leading to gout attacks.

In conclusion, for individuals experiencing joint pain, it may be beneficial to avoid or limit dairy products. This is because dairy products can promote inflammation, contribute to weight gain, and exacerbate symptoms of joint pain. It's important to speak with a healthcare provider to determine the best course of action and to also consider alternatives such as plant-based milk, soy milk, and almond milk for a healthy diet.

In addition to consuming foods that are beneficial for joint health, some people may benefit from taking dietary supplements. Some of the dietary supplements that may be beneficial for joint health include omega-3 fatty acids, glucosamine, chondroitin, and turmeric. Consuming these supplements as directed can help reduce joint pain and inflammation.

HERBAL REMEDIES

Herbal remedies have been used for centuries to treat a variety of ailments, including joint pain. Joint pain can be caused by a number of factors, including osteoarthritis, rheumatoid arthritis, and injury. Herbs can be used to reduce inflammation, improve circulation, and promote healing in the joints.

Some of the most commonly used herbs for joint pain are:

1. Turmeric

Turmeric is a popular herb that has been used for centuries in traditional medicine to treat a variety of ailments, including joint pain. The active ingredient in turmeric, curcumin, has powerful anti-inflammatory and antioxidant properties that make it an effective treatment for joint pain.

One of the main causes of joint pain is inflammation. Curcumin, the active ingredient in turmeric, has been found to reduce inflammation by inhibiting the production of inflammatory compounds in the body. This can help to reduce pain and swelling in the joints, making it an effective treatment for conditions such as osteoarthritis and rheumatoid arthritis.

In addition to its anti-inflammatory properties, curcumin is also an antioxidant. Antioxidants help to protect the body from damage caused by free radicals, which can lead to inflammation and cell damage. By protecting the joints from damage, curcumin can help to promote healing and improve joint health.

Turmeric can be consumed in several forms such as in supplement form or as a spice in food. It is also commonly used in Ayurvedic and traditional Chinese medicine to treat joint pain.

Overall, turmeric is a natural remedy that can be an effective treatment for joint pain. Its anti-inflammatory and antioxidant properties make it a powerful tool in reducing joint pain and promoting joint health. However, it is important to speak with a healthcare professional before taking turmeric supplements as they may interact with other medications.

2. ginger

Ginger is a popular spice that has been used for centuries in traditional medicine to alleviate various health conditions, including joint pain. The active compounds in ginger, such as gingerol and shogaol, have anti-inflammatory and analgesic properties that can help reduce pain and inflammation in the joints.

One way ginger may help with joint pain is by inhibiting the production of inflammatory mediators, such as prostaglandins and leukotrienes. These mediators are responsible for causing inflammation and pain in the joints, and by inhibiting their production, ginger can help reduce joint pain and inflammation.

Another way ginger may help with joint pain is by reducing oxidative stress. Oxidative stress is a condition in which the body's cells are damaged by free radicals, which can contribute to the development of joint pain and inflammation. Ginger contains antioxidants that can help protect the body's cells from free radical damage, which can help reduce joint pain and inflammation.

Ginger can also help with joint pain by improving blood circulation. Improved blood circulation can help bring more oxygen and nutrients to the joints, which can help reduce joint pain and inflammation.

There are several ways to consume ginger to alleviate joint pain. Fresh ginger root can be grated or minced and added to foods, such as stir-fries, soups, and marinades. Ginger can also be consumed as a supplement in capsule or powder form, or consumed as tea. However, it is always best to speak with a healthcare professional before starting any new supplement regimen.

Overall, ginger has been found to be an effective natural remedy for joint pain due to its anti-inflammatory and antioxidant properties. It can help reduce pain and inflammation in the joints, improve blood circulation, and protect the body's cells from free radical damage. It is a safe and natural alternative that can be consumed in various forms.

3. Boswellia

Boswellia, also known as Indian frankincense, is an herbal extract derived from the resin of the Boswellia serrata tree. It has been used for centuries in traditional Ayurvedic medicine to alleviate various health conditions, including joint pain.

Boswellia contains compounds called boswellic acids, which have anti-inflammatory and analgesic properties that can help reduce pain and inflammation in the joints. These compounds work by inhibiting the production of inflammatory mediators, such as leukotrienes, which are responsible for causing inflammation and pain in the joints. By inhibiting their production, Boswellia can help reduce joint pain and inflammation.

Boswellia may also help with joint pain by reducing oxidative stress. Oxidative stress is a condition in which the body's cells are damaged by free radicals, which can contribute to the development of joint pain and inflammation. Boswellia contains antioxidants that can help protect the body's cells from free radical damage, which can help reduce joint pain and inflammation.

Boswellia is also believed to help with joint pain by improving blood circulation. Improved blood circulation can help bring more oxygen and nutrients to the joints, which can help reduce joint pain and inflammation.

Boswellia is typically consumed as a supplement in capsule or powder form, although it is always best to speak with a healthcare professional before starting any new supplement regimen. The dosage of Boswellia may vary depending on the condition and the person's overall health.

Overall, Boswellia has been found to be an effective natural remedy for joint pain due to its anti-inflammatory and antioxidant properties. It can help reduce pain and inflammation in the joints, improve blood circulation, and protect the body's cells from free radical damage. It is a safe and natural alternative that can be consumed in supplement form. However, as with any supplement, it is important to talk to your healthcare professional before starting any new supplement regimen.

4. Devil's Claw

Devil's claw is a plant native to southern Africa that has been used for centuries in traditional medicine to alleviate various health conditions, including joint pain. The active compounds in devil's claw, such as harpagoside and beta-sitosterol, have anti-inflammatory and analgesic properties that can help reduce pain and inflammation in the joints.

One way devil's claw may help with joint pain is by inhibiting the production of inflammatory mediators, such as prostaglandins and leukotrienes. These mediators are responsible for causing inflammation and pain in the joints, and by inhibiting their production, devil's claw can help reduce joint pain and inflammation.

Devil's claw may also help with joint pain by reducing oxidative stress. Oxidative stress is a condition in which the body's cells are damaged by free radicals, which can contribute to the development of joint pain and inflammation. Devil's claw contains antioxidants that can help protect the body's cells from free radical damage, which can help reduce joint pain and inflammation.

Devil's claw is also believed to help with joint pain by improving blood circulation. Improved blood circulation can help bring more oxygen and nutrients to the joints, which can help reduce joint pain and inflammation.

Devil's claw is typically consumed as a supplement in capsule or powder form, although it is always best to speak with a healthcare professional before starting any new supplement regimen. The dosage of devil's claw may vary depending on the condition and the person's overall health.

Overall, devil's claw has been found to be an effective natural remedy for joint pain due to its anti-inflammatory and antioxidant properties. It can help reduce pain and inflammation in the joints, improve blood circulation, and protect the body's cells from free radical damage. It is a safe and natural alternative that can be consumed in supplement form. However, as with any supplement, it is important to talk to your healthcare professional before starting any new supplement regimen. Additionally, it's important to note that Devil's claw may have interactions with certain medications, such as blood thinners, so it's always better to consult with a healthcare professional before taking it.

5. Willow bark

Willow bark is derived from the bark of the white willow tree and has been used for centuries in traditional medicine to alleviate various health conditions, including joint pain.

The active compounds in willow bark, such as salicin and salicylic acid, have anti-inflammatory and analgesic properties that can help reduce pain and inflammation in the joints.

One way willow bark may help with joint pain is by inhibiting the production of inflammatory mediators, such as prostaglandins and leukotrienes. These mediators are responsible for causing inflammation and pain in the joints, and by inhibiting their production, willow bark can help reduce joint pain and inflammation.

Willow bark may also help with joint pain by reducing oxidative stress. Oxidative stress is a condition in which the body's cells are damaged by free radicals, which can contribute to the development of joint pain and inflammation. Willow bark contains antioxidants that can help protect the body's cells from free radical damage, which can help reduce joint pain and inflammation.

Willow bark can also help with joint pain by improving blood circulation. Improved blood circulation can help bring more oxygen and nutrients to the joints, which can help reduce joint pain and inflammation.

Willow bark is typically consumed as a supplement in capsule or powder form, but it can also be consumed as a tea. However, it is always best to speak with a healthcare professional before starting any new supplement regimen.

It is important to note that willow bark should not be consumed by people who are sensitive or allergic to aspirin. It can also interact with other medications such as blood thinners, so it's always better to consult with a healthcare professional before taking it.

Overall, willow bark has been found to be an effective natural remedy for joint pain due to its anti-inflammatory and antioxidant properties. It can help reduce pain and inflammation in the joints, improve blood circulation, and protect the body's cells from free radical damage. It is a natural alternative that can be consumed in supplement form or as tea. However, as with any supplement, it is important to talk to your healthcare professional before starting any new supplement regimen.

In addition to these herbs, there are many other natural remedies that may be effective in treating joint pain. For example, omega-3 fatty acids, which are found in fish oil, have been shown to reduce inflammation and improve joint health. Glucosamine and chondroitin, which are found in cartilage, may also help to improve joint health.

When using herbal remedies for joint pain, it is important to remember that they may not work for everyone. It is also important to talk to a healthcare professional before taking any new supplements, as they may interact with other medications you are taking.

In conclusion, herbal remedies can be an effective way to reduce pain and inflammation in the joints. Turmeric, ginger, Boswellia, devil's claw, and willow bark are some of the most commonly used herbs for joint pain, but there are many other natural remedies that may also be effective. It is important to talk to a healthcare professional before taking any new supplements, as they may interact with other medications you are taking.

EXERCISE

Exercise is an important aspect of maintaining overall health and well-being, and it can also play a crucial role in managing and reducing joint pain. Joint pain, which can affect any joint in the body, is a common issue that can be caused by a variety of factors, including osteoarthritis, rheumatoid arthritis, gout, and injuries. Regular exercise can help alleviate joint pain by strengthening the muscles surrounding the joint, improving flexibility and range of motion, and reducing inflammation.

Strength training is particularly effective in helping to alleviate joint pain. By strengthening the muscles surrounding the joint, weight-bearing exercises such as squats and lunges can help take pressure off the joint, reducing pain and improving function. Additionally, strength training can help improve bone density, which can be beneficial for people with conditions such as osteoarthritis. It's important to start with low weight and gradually increase the weight as your muscles get stronger.

Flexibility and range of motion exercises are also important for managing joint pain. Stretching exercises, such as yoga and tai chi, can help improve flexibility and range of motion in the affected joint, reducing stiffness and pain. Additionally, these exercises can help improve balance and coordination, which can be beneficial for people with conditions such as rheumatoid arthritis.

Cardiovascular exercises, such as walking, cycling, and swimming, can also be helpful in managing joint pain. These types of exercises can improve circulation, which can help reduce inflammation and swelling in the affected joint. Additionally, cardiovascular exercise can help to improve overall fitness and reduce the risk of obesity, which can be a contributing factor to joint pain.

Aquatic exercises, such as water aerobics, can be especially beneficial for people with joint pain. The buoyancy of the water can help to reduce pressure on the joints, making it easier to move and exercise. Additionally, the resistance provided by the water can help to improve muscle strength and flexibility.

It's important to note that while exercise can be beneficial for managing joint pain, it is important to listen to your body and not push yourself too hard. If you experience pain or discomfort during exercise, it is important to stop and speak with your doctor or physical therapist. They can help you to develop a safe and effective exercise plan that is tailored to your specific needs and limitations.

In addition to exercise, there are other lifestyle changes that can help to alleviate joint pain. Maintaining a healthy weight, eating a well-balanced diet, and getting enough sleep can all help to reduce inflammation and improve overall health. Additionally, it is important to avoid smoking and limit alcohol consumption, as these can contribute to joint pain and inflammation.

In conclusion, regular exercise can be an effective tool for managing and reducing joint pain. By strengthening the muscles surrounding the joint, improving flexibility and range of motion, and reducing inflammation, exercise can help to alleviate pain and improve function. It's important to listen to your body and not push yourself too hard, and to work with your doctor or physical therapist to develop a safe and effective exercise plan. Along with exercise, maintaining a healthy weight, eating a well-balanced diet, getting enough sleep, avoiding smoking, and limiting alcohol consumption can also help to alleviate joint pain.

STRESS MANAGEMENT

Stress can have a significant impact on overall health and well-being, and it can also contribute to joint pain. Stress can cause muscle tension and inflammation, which can exacerbate joint pain and make it more difficult to manage. Stress management techniques, such as relaxation techniques, exercise, and therapy, can help to alleviate joint pain by reducing muscle tension and inflammation.

Relaxation techniques, such as deep breathing, meditation, and yoga, can help to reduce muscle tension and inflammation by promoting relaxation and reducing the body's stress response. These techniques can also help to improve sleep quality, which can be beneficial for managing joint pain.

Exercise is also an effective stress management technique and can also help to alleviate joint pain. Regular physical activity can help to reduce muscle tension and inflammation, and improve overall fitness and well-being. However, it's important to choose exercises that are low-impact and easy on the joints, such as swimming, cycling, and yoga.

Cognitive-behavioral therapy (CBT) and other forms of therapy can also be beneficial for managing stress and joint pain. Therapy can help individuals to identify and change negative thought patterns and behaviors that may be contributing to their stress and pain. It can also help to develop coping strategies and stress management techniques, such as relaxation techniques and exercise.

In addition to these stress management techniques, other lifestyle changes can also help to alleviate joint pain caused by stress. Maintaining a healthy diet, getting enough sleep, and avoiding smoking and excessive alcohol consumption can all help to reduce inflammation and improve overall health.

In conclusion, stress management techniques can be an effective tool for managing and reducing joint pain. Relaxation techniques, exercise, and therapy can help to reduce muscle tension and inflammation, which can exacerbate joint pain. In addition to these stress management techniques, other lifestyle changes such as maintaining a healthy diet, getting enough sleep, and avoiding smoking and excessive alcohol consumption can also help to alleviate joint pain caused by stress. It's important to work with a healthcare professional to develop a comprehensive plan that addresses both the physical and emotional aspects of joint pain.

CHAPTER THREE

ADDITIONAL CONSIDERATIONS

ESSENTIAL OILS

Since ancient times, essential oils have been utilized as herbal treatments for a variety of illnesses, including joint discomfort. Joint pain may vary from slight discomfort to severe pain and stiffness and can be brought on by a number of conditions, including arthritis, injury, or overuse. The anti-inflammatory, analgesic, and antioxidant qualities of essential oils may aid in reducing joint discomfort and enhancing joint mobility.

Ginger oil is one of the most well-liked essential oils for joint discomfort. Ginger includes substances with anti-inflammatory and pain-relieving effects known as gingerols and shogaols. These substances aid in reducing joint swelling and inflammation, which may lessen discomfort and increase mobility.

Turmeric oil is another well-liked essential oil for arthritic pain. Curcumin, a substance found in turmeric, has both anti-inflammatory and antioxidant effects. Because of its ability to lessen joint pain and inflammation, curcumin may also be able to halt the course of certain forms of arthritis.

Joint discomfort may also be treated with peppermint oil. Menthol, which has a cooling impact on the skin and may help to lessen joint discomfort and inflammation, is a component of peppermint. Additionally, it is believed that peppermint oil stimulates blood flow, which might lessen joint inflammation and stiffness.

Additionally used for joint discomfort, is eucalyptus oil. Eucalyptus includes substances with anti-inflammatory and pain-relieving effects termed eucalyptol and cineole. Additionally, eucalyptus oil may increase circulation and lessen inflammation, which helps lessen joint discomfort and increase mobility.

For joint discomfort, cedarwood oil is also used. Because of its anti-inflammatory and pain-relieving qualities, cedarwood oil is employed. Additionally, it's believed that cedarwood oil increases circulation and lowers inflammation, which may aid to lessen joint discomfort and increase mobility.

Joint discomfort may also be treated with frankincense oil. Due to its anti-inflammatory and pain-relieving qualities, frankincense oil is employed. Additionally, it is believed that frankincense oil increases circulation and lowers inflammation, which may help to lessen joint discomfort and increase mobility.

Being extremely concentrated and having the potential to cause skin irritation or allergic responses in some people, essential oils should be used with care. Before applying an essential oil to the skin, it is usually advised to dilute it with carrier oil. Additionally, it is best to see a doctor before taking any essential oils and they should never be used without competent medical supervision.

In conclusion, using essential oils as a treatment for joint discomfort may be safe and helpful. It is crucial to utilize them cautiously and under a healthcare professional's supervision. With their anti-inflammatory and painkilling characteristics, essential oils including frankincense, ginger, turmeric, peppermint, eucalyptus, and cedarwood may help to lessen joint pain and increase mobility. Before using any essential oil, a patch test should always be performed, and medical advice should always be sought.

ACUPUNCTURE

Acupoints are precise points on the body where small needles are inserted during acupuncture, a kind of traditional Chinese medicine. It is said to promote healing by balancing the body's Qi, or energy, flow. Since ancient times, acupuncture has been used to treat a wide range of illnesses, including joint pain.

A number of conditions, including arthritis, trauma, or overuse, may result in joint discomfort. By enhancing Qi and blood flow, lowering inflammation, and encouraging the body's natural pain-relieving chemical, endorphin synthesis, acupuncture may assist to lessen joint discomfort and increase joint mobility.

Acupoints in the body that correspond to the injured joint are stimulated by acupuncture. These spots are said to regulate the local blood and qi flow, which helps lessen pain and inflammation. Additionally, acupuncture may promote the release of endorphins, which can lessen pain and enhance general well-being.

Additionally, acupuncture has been shown to increase circulation and lessen muscular tension, which may assist to lessen joint edema and stiffness. Enhancing flexibility and range of motion may also aid in enhancing joint mobility.

To increase the efficacy of the therapy, other acupuncture methods, like Cupping, Moxibustion, and Gua Sha, may be employed in addition to the insertion of needles.

It is essential to remember that when done by a trained professional, acupuncture is usually regarded as safe. However, there is always a chance of difficulties and adverse effects with any medical procedure. It is advised to seek out a qualified acupuncturist who is licensed and has the required education, training, and experience.

Finally, acupuncture is a secure and reliable method of treating joint discomfort. It may aid in pain relief, increased joint mobility, and general well-being. The damaged joint's precise acupoints on the body are stimulated by acupuncture, which also encourages blood and Qi flow, reduces inflammation, and increases endorphin synthesis. It is usually advised to find a certified acupuncturist before beginning the procedure.

SUPPLEMENTS

Many individuals have joint discomfort, which is a typical issue, especially as they become older. Joint pain may be brought on by a number of factors, including trauma, inflammation, and degenerative diseases like osteoarthritis. While numerous prescription drugs are available to alleviate joint pain, there are also a variety of dietary supplements that promise to be effective.

Two of the most well-known supplements for joint discomfort are glucosamine and chondroitin. A naturally occurring substance called glucosamine is utilized to create and repair cartilage, the tissue that cushions the joints. A similar Substance, chondroitin, supports cartilage's flexibility and durability. Together, these vitamins may lessen joint discomfort and inflammation while also delaying the onset of osteoarthritis and other degenerative disorders.

Omega-3 fatty acids are another dietary supplement that can be beneficial for joint discomfort. These good fats, which are included in fish oil, have been demonstrated to have anti-inflammatory effects. They might enhance overall joint health and lessen joint pain and inflammation.

Boswellia sometimes referred to as Indian frankincense, is a kind of tree resin that has been used for millennia in

Ayurvedic medicine to treat a number of ailments, including joint discomfort. Boswellia's main ingredients, known as Boswellia, have analgesic and anti-inflammatory qualities that may aid to lessen pain and inflammation in the joints.

Spices like turmeric are often seen in Indian and Southeast Asian dishes. Traditional medicine also uses it for a number of ailments, such as joint discomfort. Curcumin, the main ingredient in turmeric, has anti-inflammatory and antioxidant qualities that may aid to lessen joint discomfort and inflammation.

Additionally, for millennia, supplements like white willow bark, ginger, and devil's claw have been used to relieve joint pain. White willow bark contains substances called salicin, which are comparable to the main element in aspirin and may be used to relieve pain and inflammation. Devil's claw

is an ancient African cure that has anti-inflammatory effects.
Ginger is a natural anti-inflammatory and antioxidant.

While supplements may be a helpful complement to a strategy for treating joint pain, it's vital to remember that they shouldn't be taken in lieu of traditional medical therapy. The best course of action is to speak with a healthcare professional before beginning a new supplement regimen. Self-diagnosis and self-treatment may sometimes result in major health problems.

In summary, there are several substances that might ease joint discomfort. Supplements that have been used to treat joint pain include glucosamine and chondroitin, omega-3 fatty acids, boswellia, turmeric, devil's claw, ginger, and white willow bark. These substances have been shown to have anti-inflammatory and pain-relieving qualities. However, it's crucial to get medical advice before beginning any new supplement regimen and to avoid using supplements in lieu of regular medical treatment.

PROFESSIONAL CARE

There are many different reasons of joint pain, including injury, inflammation, and degenerative disorders like osteoarthritis. Joint pain is a widespread issue that many individuals experience. Even though there are several over-the-counter medications that may be used to alleviate joint pain, it is often preferable to seek expert treatment in order to correctly identify and treat the underlying disease.

A primary care physician or a specialist, such as an orthopedic surgeon or rheumatologist, may assist in identifying the source of joint pain and developing a treatment strategy. To diagnose the ailment, a physical examination, a medical history, and imaging tests like X-rays or MRI may be ordered.

The healthcare professional may suggest a number of therapy choices after determining the reason for the joint discomfort. For instance, if osteoarthritis is the source of the joint pain, they may advise a mix of physical therapy, healthy eating habits, and medicine to lessen pain and inflammation, such as non-steroidal anti-inflammatory drugs (NSAIDs) or disease-modifying anti-rheumatic drugs (DMARDS).

An essential part of treating joint discomfort is physical therapy. Exercises that serve to increase the range of motion, flexibility, and strength in the injured joint may be taught to patients by physical therapists. To aid with pain relief and enhance mobility, they could also advise using aids like canes or braces.

Affected joint discomfort and inflammation may also be treated with injections like corticosteroids or hyaluronic acid. In order to relieve pain, corticosteroids, which are potent anti-inflammatory drugs, are injected directly into the joint. The body naturally produces hyaluronic acid, which is utilized to lubricate and cushion the joints. Hyaluronic acid injections may be used to ease discomfort and enhance joint function.

When non-invasive therapies do not relieve joint discomfort, surgery may be an alternative. A frequent surgical treatment is a joint replacement, which involves removing the injured joint and replacing it with a synthetic one composed of metal or plastic. Patients with severe joint injury may get considerable pain alleviation and improved mobility after this procedure.

Maintaining a healthy lifestyle is crucial to managing joint pain in addition to these therapeutic choices. Reduced joint stress and improve overall joint health may be achieved by a good diet, consistent exercise, and keeping a healthy weight.

In conclusion, receiving competent treatment is essential for treating joint discomfort. A primary care physician or a specialist, such as an orthopedic surgeon or rheumatologist, may assist in making a diagnosis and developing a treatment strategy. Surgery, medicine, physical therapy, and injections are all available as treatments. In order to manage joint discomfort, it's crucial to keep a healthy lifestyle. It's always advisable to seek expert care since doing self-diagnosis and self-treatment might result in major health issues.

CONCLUSION

Finally, joint pain is a frequent condition that may have a big influence on a person's quality of life. Injury, inflammation, and arthritis are just a few of the causes of joint pain. Understanding the underlying causes of joint pain is crucial for finding a cure.

Herbal medicines, food and nutrition, exercise, and stress reduction are just a few of the natural therapies that may be utilized to treat joint pain. Herbal medicines with anti-inflammatory and pain-relieving characteristics include turmeric, ginger, bromelain, Boswellia, and curcumin. These herbs may be taken as supplements or as an ingredient in food and beverages.

The management of joint pain also heavily depends on diet and nutrition. It is possible to lessen inflammation and ease joint pain by eating a diet high in anti-inflammatory foods including fish, nuts, fruits, and vegetables. Fish like salmon, which contain omega-3 fatty acids, may be very helpful for treating joint discomfort.

Another crucial component of controlling joint discomfort is exercise. The muscles around the joint may be strengthened by regular exercise, which can help to lessen discomfort and increase mobility. For those with joint discomfort, low-impact activities like swimming, bicycling, and yoga are very helpful.

An essential component of controlling joint pain is stress management. Joint pain may become more intense as a result of increased inflammatory chemical production brought on by stress. Joint discomfort may be eased by engaging in stress-relieving activities like yoga, deep breathing exercises, and meditation.

There are various more factors to take into account in addition to the natural therapies mentioned above for controlling joint pain. Applying peppermint, ginger, and turmeric essential oils topically helps ease pain and inflammation. Another complementary treatment that may be used to treat joint discomfort is acupuncture. To maintain joint health, supplements like glucosamine and chondroitin are also an option.

Finally, it's crucial to get medical advice before attempting any novel natural treatments for joint pain. Joint pain may be reduced and general joint health can be enhanced with the appropriate natural treatments and lifestyle modifications. It's also crucial to remember that although natural treatments might ease joint discomfort, they shouldn't be utilized in place of medical attention. It's crucial to get medical help if joint discomfort continues or worsens.

In conclusion, controlling joint pain may be a challenging task, but with the correct natural treatments and dietary adjustments, joint pain can be reduced and overall joint health can be enhanced. Before attempting any novel natural treatments for joint pain, it's crucial to speak with a healthcare practitioner. If joint pain continues or worsens, you should also contact a doctor. Living pain-free and taking part in all your favorite activities is feasible with the appropriate strategy.

9 798375 174983